Cannabis Fit

The Health Enthusiast's Guide to Infused Nutrition and Fitness

By

Vanessa S. Castaneda

Table of Contents

Introduction

In recent years, the nexus of cannabis, health, and fitness has risen from the margins to the forefront of wellness culture. As public attitudes change and scientific research advances, the incorporation of cannabis into health and fitness routines becomes more acceptable and recognized. This article seeks to refute popular fallacies about cannabis use in fitness and nutrition, shedding light on its numerous benefits when used carefully and thoughtfully.

Cannabis, a plant with complicated biochemistry, provides more than just recreational benefits. Among its various constituents, cannabinoids like CBD (cannabidiol) and THC (tetrahydrocannabinol) are notable for their medicinal and nutritional properties. CBD, known for its anti-inflammatory characteristics and absence of euphoric effects, has gained popularity in health circles for stress relief, rehabilitation, and pain treatment. THC, while psychotropic, is praised for its ability to relieve pain, promote hunger, and improve sleep. These cannabinoids, along with others like CBG (cannabigerol) and CBN (cannabinol), function in tandem through the entourage effect, improving the body's ability to heal, recover, and perform.

The nutritional composition of cannabis itself should not be neglected. Hemp seeds, which come from the same cannabis plant, are high in protein, vital fatty acids, and minerals, making them a superfood in and of themselves. When used with a well-balanced diet, cannabis can benefit not only physical but also mental health by reducing stress and increasing sleep patterns, all of which are essential for recovery and exercise performance.

This guide will lead you through the changing landscape of cannabis in health and fitness, providing insights on how to incorporate this ancient plant into current wellness practices. By knowing the science underlying cannabis and its effects on the body, readers will be able to make informed decisions about adding it to their health and fitness routines, unlocking new levels of well-being and energy. Through this examination, we hope to change people's attitudes about cannabis, demonstrating its potential as a beneficial ally in accomplishing health and fitness goals. Join us on a journey into the realm of cannabis-infused nutrition and fitness, where wellness meets nature's richness.

Chapter 1

Cannabis and Nutrition

Understanding cannabis' nutritional profile is important as we work to incorporate it into our health and wellness regimens. Cannabis, while frequently viewed through the lens of its euphoric qualities, contains a plethora of nutritional benefits that can play an important role in a well-balanced diet and healthy metabolism.

Understanding Cannabis's Nutritional Profile

Cannabis, particularly in its non-psychoactive variants such as hemp, is an extremely nutritious plant. Hemp seeds, for example, are high in important fatty acids, including omega-3 and omega-6, in a proportion that is extremely helpful to cardiovascular health. They are also an excellent source of protein, as they contain all nine essential amino acids, making them a complete protein source, which is unusual in the plant kingdom. Hemp seeds also include fiber, vitamins, and minerals such as vitamin E, phosphorus, potassium, sodium, magnesium, sulfur, calcium, iron, and zinc.

Aside from the seeds, the leaves of the cannabis plant can be consumed in a variety of ways, such as in drinks and salads, and are rich in vitamins and antioxidants. These components can help to reduce inflammation and protect the body from the oxidative stress that many chronic diseases are connected with.

Cannabis's Role in Promoting a Healthy Diet and Metabolism

Cannabis consumption can improve health and metabolism in a variety of ways. The high fiber content of hemp seeds and leaves can improve digestion and build a healthy gut microbiota, which is essential for overall health and efficient metabolism. The essential fatty acids present in hemp seeds have been shown to promote heart health by decreasing blood pressure, lipid levels, and the risk of heart disease.

Cannabinoids, such as CBD, have been proven to directly alter metabolism. According to studies, CBD can aid in "browning" fat cells, transforming them from energy-storing white fat to energy-burning brown fat, which could benefit weight management and minimize the risks associated with metabolic syndrome.

Guidelines for Integrating Cannabis into a Balanced Diet

I. **Start with Hemp Seeds**: hemp seeds are a simple means to incorporate cannabis into your diet. They bring a nutty flavor and nutritious boost to salads, smoothies, and muesli.

II. **Consider CBD Pills**: For individuals seeking the metabolic and anti-inflammatory advantages of cannabis without the euphoric effects, CBD oil or pills can be an excellent addition. Start with minimal doses and consult with your healthcare practitioner to adapt them to your specific wellness goals.

III. **Use Whole Plant Options**: Adding whole plant choices, such as cannabis leaves, to juices or salads can bring additional nutrients and advantages. This method recognizes the plant's inherent complexity and the synergistic impact of its chemicals.

IV. **Balanced Approach**: Whenever you incorporate cannabis, make sure to take your food and lifestyle into full account. Rather than taking the place of a diet high in fruits, vegetables, lean proteins, and whole grains, it should be used in addition to them.

V. **Legal and Quality Considerations**: Be aware of the legal status of cannabis products in your area and choose high-quality, lab-tested products from trustworthy suppliers to assure safety and efficacy.

Chapter 2

Cannabis-Infused Superfoods

This chapter explores recipes that combine the nutritional powerhouse of cannabis with other superfoods, creating delicious, nutrient-dense meals that fuel the body and mind. Combining cannabis and superfoods can amplify their respective health benefits, offering a potent synergy that supports optimal health, wellness, and vitality.

Recipes for smoothies, salads, and bowls containing cannabis and other superfoods.

Cannabis-infused Green Superfood Smoothie

Ingredients:

- 1 cup spinach (high in vitamins and minerals)
- 1/2 avocado (high in healthy fats and fiber)

- 1/2 cup pineapple chunks (high in enzymes and antioxidants).
- 1 tablespoon chia seeds (high in omega-3 fatty acids and fiber)
- 1 teaspoon CBD oil
- 1 cup coconut water ice cubes (optional)

Instructions: Combine spinach, avocado, pineapple chunks, chia seeds, and CBD oil until smooth, blend in the coconut water until thoroughly combined, to adjust thickness, add ice cubes. Pour into a glass and enjoy this nutrient-dense green smoothie.

Cannabis-Infused Quinoa Superfood Salad

Ingredients:

- 1 cup cooked quinoa (full protein source)
- 1/2 cup halved cherry tomatoes (source of vitamin C and potassium).
- 1/4 cup sliced cucumber (for hydration and vitamins)
- 1/4 cup chopped red bell pepper (for antioxidants)

- 2 tablespoons pumpkin seeds (rich in zinc and magnesium)
- 1 tablespoon hemp seeds
- Cannabis-infused olive oil (dosage based on preference and legal restrictions).
- Lemon juice, salt, and pepper to taste.

Instruction: In a bowl, mix cooked quinoa, cherry tomatoes, cucumber, red bell pepper, pumpkin seeds, and hemp seeds, drizzle with cannabis-infused olive oil, and pour lemon juice over the salad, season with salt and pepper to taste, mix everything thoroughly. Serve it as a nutritious side dish or light supper.

Cannabis-Infused Acai Superfood Bowl

Ingredients:

- 1 packet frozen acai berry puree (antioxidants and heart health)
- 1 banana (potassium and energy)
- 1/2 cup mixed berries (vitamin C and fiber)

- 1 tablespoon almond butter (healthy fats and protein)
- 1 teaspoon CBD oil Toppings include sliced strawberries, granola, coconut flakes, and a drizzle of cannabis-infused honey.

Instructions: Blend the acai puree, banana, mixed berries, almond butter, and CBD oil until creamy, and transfer the mixture to a bowl, finish with sliced strawberries, granola, coconut flakes, and cannabis-infused honey. Enjoy this tasty and nutrient-dense acai bowl for breakfast or as a healthy snack.

Synergistic Effects of Combining Cannabis with Nutrient-Dense Foods for Optimal Health.

The combination of cannabis and nutrient-dense foods can provide a synergistic effect that is greater than the sum of their benefits. This symbiotic interaction improves the overall nutritional profile and health effects. Here's a discussion of how this synergy works:

Increased Nutrient Absorption:

- Cannabis compounds, including CBD and THC, have been demonstrated to improve nutritional absorption. Avocados, almonds, and olive oil provide healthy fats, which can act as transporters for cannabinoids, improving their bioavailability and effectiveness in the body.

Anti-Inflammatory Powerhouse:

- Nutrient-dense foods, such as leafy greens, berries, and seeds, are known to have anti-inflammatory qualities. When coupled with cannabinoids, particularly CBD, the anti-inflammatory effects can be enhanced. This synergy may help to lower inflammation throughout the body, aiding disorders including arthritis and inflammatory diseases.

Balanced Blood Sugar Levels:

- Whole grains, like quinoa, and a fiber-rich diet help stabilize blood sugar levels. Combining these with cannabis, which has shown promise in lowering insulin and glucose levels, could result in a more balanced approach to blood sugar management. This could be especially advantageous for diabetics or those looking for consistent energy levels.

Optimised Digestive Health:

- Consuming high-fiber foods, such as salads and bowls, promotes digestive health. Cannabis, in turn, has been linked to improved gut function and health. The combination may aid digestion, vitamin absorption, and a healthy microbiome.

Cannabinoid Receptor Activation:

- Nutrient-dense foods may affect the endocannabinoid system, which interacts with cannabinoids. This interaction can boost the effects of cannabinoids like

THC and CBD, resulting in a greater sense of well-being and balance.

Comprehensive Antioxidant Protection:

- Superfoods are frequently high in antioxidants, which help to battle oxidative stress and prevent cellular damage. Cannabis, with its antioxidant characteristics, can supplement this defense mechanism. The combined effect may lead to increased cellular health and a lower risk of chronic diseases.

Mood and Stress Management:

- Nutrients such as omega-3 fatty acids in chia seed or hemp seed can help regulate mood. Combining these nutrient-dense meals with cannabis, particularly strains with balanced CBD and THC ratios, may help to reduce stress and enhance mood.

The Holistic Wellness Approach:

- The combination of cannabis and nutrient-dense foods promotes a comprehensive approach to health. Rather than focusing on a single area of health, this synergy tackles several aspects at once, improving physical, mental, and emotional well-being.

Chapter 3

Cannabis Recipes for Pre and Post-Workout

Fitness enthusiasts are discovering the potential benefits of integrating cannabis into their workouts, which opens up a new level of support for pain relief, reduced inflammation, and improved muscle recovery. This chapter delves into the benefits of cannabis for fitness and offers tempting recipes for pre-workout energy boosts and post-workout rehabilitation.

Benefits of Cannabis in Fitness Routines

- **Pain Relief**: Cannabinoids, specifically CBD, have analgesic effects that can relieve exercise-induced pain. This natural pain reduction technique might improve the overall workout and recovery process.
- **Reduced Inflammation**: Cannabis has anti-inflammatory properties that may help reduce inflammation from physical

exertion. This can lead to a faster recovery and less muscular discomfort.

- **Muscle Recovery**: The endocannabinoid system promotes muscle recovery and repair. Cannabis, by interacting with this system, may promote muscle tissue regeneration, resulting in faster recuperation after exercises.

Pre-Workout Energy Boost: Cannabis-Infused Green Smoothie

Ingredients:

- 1 cup kale or spinach (vitamin and mineral-rich);
- 1/2 banana (natural energy source and potassium);
- 1/4 cup Greek yogurt
- 1 tablespoon almond butter, 1 teaspoon cannabis-infused honey, 1 cup coconut water, and optional ice cubes.

Instructions: Blend kale or spinach, banana, Greek yogurt, almond butter, cannabis-infused honey, and coconut water until smooth, add ice cubes for a refreshing texture. Pour into a glass and consume 30–60 minutes before your activity to get a nutrient-dense energy boost.

Post-Workout Recovery: CBD-Infused Protein Bars

Ingredients:

- 1 cup rolled oats (complex carbs)
- 1/2 cup almond butter (protein and healthy fats)
- 1/4 cup honey or maple syrup
- 1/4 cup chocolate protein powder.
- 1/4 cup chopped nuts (almonds or walnuts),
- 1 teaspoon cannabis-infused coconut oil,
- 1/2 teaspoon vanilla extract, and a pinch of sea salt.

Instructions: In a bowl, combine rolled oats, almond butter, honey or maple syrup, chocolate protein powder, chopped almonds, cannabis-infused coconut oil, vanilla essence, and sea salt, place the mixture in a lined baking dish and chill for at least 1 hour. Once firm, cut into bars for a quick and delicious post-workout snack.

Light Post-Workout Meal: Cannabis-infused Quinoa Bowl

Ingredients:

- 1 cup cooked quinoa (complete protein)
- Grilled chicken or tofu (for protein)
- Mixed veggies (broccoli, bell peppers, and cherry tomatoes)
- 1 tablespoon of cannabis-infused olive oil
- Lemon juice, salt, and pepper to taste
- Optional: avocado slices for healthy fats

Instructions: Combine cooked quinoa, grilled chicken or tofu, and mixed vegetables in a bowl, add cannabis-infused olive oil and fresh lemon juice to the bowl, season with salt and pepper to taste, (Optional)Top with avocado slices. Enjoy as a balanced post-workout meal to restore nutrients and aid with recovery.

Chapter 4

Mindfulness and Recovery

Incorporating cannabis into mindfulness techniques like yoga and meditation can improve the experience by promoting mental wellness and relaxation. This chapter delves into the relationship between cannabis and mindfulness, including recipes for teas, infusions, and light snacks that promote relaxation and mental clarity.

Enhancing Mindfulness Practices with Cannabis for Mental Health.

Integrating cannabis with mindfulness activities, particularly yoga and meditation, can provide a unique way to improve mental health. Here's an exploration of how cannabis can help promote well-being during certain practices;

1. **Stress Reduction**: Cannabis products with balanced CBD and THC concentrations have been linked to

reduced stress levels. When used with mindfulness activities, it may promote a deeper state of relaxation, allowing people to better manage stress and anxiety.

2. **Increased Sensory Awareness**: Cannabis usage can improve sensory perception, making yoga and meditation more immersive. This increased awareness may result in a stronger connection to the body, breath, and environment, generating a sense of presence.

3. **Improved Mind-Body Connection**: CBD can enhance mindfulness activities by increasing awareness of the body. This stronger mind-body connection can improve the overall experience by allowing for a better understanding and acceptance of one's physical and mental states.

4. **Enhanced Focus and Concentration**: Cannabis strains with high CBD levels have been shown to improve focus and concentration. For those who meditate, this can help them retain a clear and

concentrated mind, allowing for a deeper contemplative experience.

5. **Relaxation and Release of Tension**: Cannabis can help relax muscles and relieve physical strain. This can be especially useful in yoga practices, where bodily relaxation is typically an important component. The combination of cannabis and yoga may result in a deeper sense of relaxation and flexibility.

6. **Facilitation of Mindfulness and States**: Cannabis can cause altered states of consciousness, which can facilitate the entry of people into mindfulness and meditation states. Some may experience a deeper level of awareness of themselves and their surroundings through these techniques as a result of this.

Tips for Incorporating Cannabis into Mindfulness Practice

I. **Mindful Dosing**: Begin with low dosages and progressively increase until you reach the level that complements your practice without overpowering it.

II. **Choose the Right Strain**: Strains with balanced CBD and THC content, or higher CBD content, are frequently advised for mindfulness activities because they induce calm without producing strong psychoactive effects.

III. **Respect Individual Tolerance**: Everyone reacts differently to cannabis. Respect your tolerance levels and be aware of the impacts on your body and mind.

IV. **Experiment Mindfully**: Recognise that cannabis' effects might vary, so approach experimenting with an open mind. Pay close attention to how it affects your mental and physical states during and after mindfulness exercises.

V. **Legal Points to Remember**: Make certain the way you consume cannabis complies with applicable local laws and regulations.

Recipes for Teas, Infusion, and Light Snacks that Promote Leisure and Mental Clarity.

Cannabis-infused lavender Chamomile Tea

Ingredients:

- 1 tablespoon dried lavender flowers
- 1 tablespoon dried chamomile flowers
- 1 teaspoon cannabis-infused honey
- 1 cup hot water.

Instructions: To prepare, add lavender and chamomile flowers to a tea infuser, allow the herbs to steep in boiling water for 5–7 minutes, remove the infuser, and add cannabis-infused honey. Sip carefully and relish the calming effects of this delicious tea.

CBD-infused Citrus Mint Infusion

Ingredients:

- 1 green tea bag
- 1 sprig of fresh mint
- 1/2 teaspoon CBD oil

- Slices of orange or lemon
- 1 cup of boiling water

Instructions: Steep the green tea bag and fresh mint in boiling water for 3–5 minutes, remove the tea bag and stir in the CBD oil, garnish with orange or lemon slices. This delicious beverage promotes mental clarity and relaxation.

Cannabis-infused Almond Butter and Banana Rice Cakes

Ingredients:

- Rice cakes
- Almond butter
- Sliced banana
- Cannabis-infused coconut oil
- Optional, a sprinkle of cinnamon.

Instructions: Spread almond butter on rice cake, Top with a banana, sliced, and sprinkle with cannabis-infused coconut oil, (Optional) Sprinkle with cinnamon for extra flavor. Enjoy this light and tasty snack to give you a boost of energy while practicing mindfulness.

Blueberry CBD Bliss Balls

Ingredients:

- 1 cup of dried blueberries
- 1 cup of almonds
- 1 tablespoon of chia seeds
- 1 tablespoon of CBD-infused honey
- 1/2 teaspoon vanilla extract
- Optional: shredded coconut for rolling.

Instructions: In a food processor, combine dried blueberries, almonds, chia seeds, CBD-infused honey, and vanilla essence to make a sticky dough. Shape the mixture into tiny balls, Roll the balls in shredded coconut for extra texture, Refrigerate for at least 30 minutes before serving. These happiness balls are a healthy and convenient snack for relaxation and mental clarity.

Minty CBD Avocado Citrus Salad

Ingredients:

- Mixed greens (arugula, spinach)

- 1 ripe avocado, sliced
- Grapefruit segments
- 1 tablespoon chopped fresh mint

Dressing: 1 tablespoon of CBD-infused olive oil, 1 tablespoon of citrus juice, salt, and pepper to taste.

Instructions: Place mixed greens on a plate, Top with sliced avocado and grapefruit segments, Add fresh mint to the salad. To prepare the dressing, combine CBD-infused olive oil, citrus juice, salt, and pepper in a small bowl. Drizzle the dressing on the salad for a refreshing and mentally invigorating combo.

Chapter 5

Weight Management and Cannabis

Understanding cannabis's impacts on appetite and metabolism is crucial for unlocking its promise in weight management. This chapter looks into the role of cannabis in these areas and presents low-calorie, nutrient-dense meals specifically designed for people looking to lose weight with cannabis.

The Role of Cannabis in Appetite Control and Metabolism

Cannabis, with its varied array of cannabinoids, has sparked interest due to its possible impact on appetite management and metabolism. Here's an investigation into the present understanding in these areas:

1. **Appetite Control**

   - **THC and Appetite Stimulation**: Tetrahydrocannabinol (THC), one of the principal cannabinoids in cannabis, is well-known for its appetite-stimulating properties, sometimes known as "the munchies." It interacts with the endocannabinoid system, primarily the brain's CB1 receptors, causing the production of hunger-inducing chemicals.

- **CBD and Appetite Regulation**: Cannabidiol (CBD), a key cannabinoid, has a complex link with appetite regulation. While some studies indicate that it may impact hunger, the effects are not as clear as those of THC. CBD may interact with CB1 receptors in a way that does not regularly generate hunger, making it a viable choice for appetite regulation without considerable stimulation.

- **The Endocannabinoid System (ECS)**: The endocannabinoid system is essential for hunger control. It is made up of cannabinoids, receptors (CB1 and CB2), and enzymes. THC's interaction with CB1 receptors in the brain's hypothalamus contributes to increased hunger, while CBD's interaction with the receptors may moderate appetite signals.

2. Metabolism

- **CBD's Metabolic Effects**: New research indicates that CBD may have metabolic benefits. It has the potential to alter several areas of metabolism, including fat browning. Fat browning is the process of transforming white adipose tissue (WAT), which stores energy, to brown adipose tissue (BAT), which burns calories. This process has consequences for both weight management and metabolic health.
- **Energy Expenditure and Thermogenesis**: Some studies suggest that cannabinoids, particularly CBD, may impact metabolic processes such as energy consumption and thermogenesis. These impacts could perhaps help achieve a more balanced metabolic state.
- **Possible Effects on Insulin Sensitivity:** According to research, cannabis may help

improve insulin sensitivity. Improved insulin sensitivity is connected with better glucose metabolism, which lowers the risk of metabolic diseases such as type 2 diabetes.

3. Personal Variability

- **Individual Reactions**: It's important to understand that different people react to cannabis in different ways. The way that an individual perceives the impacts on hunger and metabolism depends on several factors, including heredity, tolerance, and general health.
- **Dose-Dependent Effects**: Cannabis' effects on hunger and metabolism are frequently dose-dependent. Low to moderate doses may provide different results than higher ones, and striking the appropriate balance is critical to minimizing any adverse effects.

4. Weight Management Considerations

- **Balance THC and CBD**: For those interested in the potential advantages of cannabis for weight loss, achieving a balance of THC and CBD concentrations in strains or products may be critical. CBD-dominant strains or products may be preferable for those looking for hunger control without excessive excitement.
- **Diet and Lifestyle Factors**: It's crucial to understand that cannabis alone isn't a miracle cure for weight loss. A comprehensive approach that includes a balanced diet, regular exercise, and a healthy lifestyle is essential for general health.

Low-calorie, Nutrient-Dense Cannabis-Infused Meals for Weight Management

Cannabis-infused Green Detox Smoothie:

Ingredients:

- 1 cup kale or spinach

- 1/2 cucumber
- 1/2 green apple
- 1/2 juiced lemon
- 1 teaspoon cannabis-infused olive oil
- 1 cup water or coconut water
- Ice cubes (optional)

Instructions: Blend kale or spinach with cucumber, green apple, lemon juice, cannabis-infused olive oil, and water until smooth. Add ice cubes for a refreshing texture. This nutrient-dense, low-calorie smoothie provides a delicious and hydrating experience.

Pesto with CBD-Infused Zucchini Noodles

Ingredients:

- Zucchini noodles
- Halved cherry tomatoes
- Pine nuts
- Fresh basil leaves
- 1 tablespoon CBD-infused olive oil
- Minced garlic
- Salt and pepper to taste.

Instructions: In a skillet, sauté minced garlic in CBD-infused olive oil until fragrant. Combine the zucchini noodles, cherry tomatoes, and pine nuts.

Cook until zucchini noodles are soft. Combine with fresh basil leaves, salt, and pepper. This light and tasty dish is ideal for a low-calorie, CBD-infused meal.

Cannabis-infused Chia Seed Pudding

Ingredients:

- 2 tbsp chia seeds
- 1 cup almond milk
- 1 tsp cannabis-infused honey
- Fresh berries on top

Instructions: Combine chia seeds, almond milk, and cannabis-infused honey in a jar. Stir thoroughly and chill for at least 2 hours or overnight. Garnish with fresh berries before serving. This chia seed pudding is a nutritious and low-calorie snack or breakfast.

CBD-infused Grilled Vegetable Salad

Ingredients:

- Grilled vegetables (zucchini, bell peppers, asparagus),
- Cooked quinoa
- 1 tablespoon CBD-infused balsamic vinaigrette, fresh herbs (parsley, mint),
- Lemon zest
- Salt, and pepper to taste.

Instructions: Mix grilled vegetables and cooked quinoa in a bowl, drizzle CBD-infused balsamic vinaigrette on the salad, and mix in fresh herbs, lemon zest, salt, and pepper. This colorful salad is a nutrient-dense, CBD-infused option for a filling and light supper.

Cannabis-Infused Minty Green Tea

Ingredients:

- 1 green tea bag
- Fresh mint leaves
- 1 teaspoon of cannabis-infused honey
- Lemon slices
- 1 cup of boiling water

Instructions: Steep the green tea bag and fresh mint leaves in boiling water for 3–5 minutes, remove the tea bag, and add cannabis-infused honey, garnish with lemon slices. This soothing tea is a delicious, low-calorie way to promote relaxation and weight management.

Chapter 6

Customizing Your Cannabis Diet

Customizing cannabis-infused meals to meet specific nutritional demands provides a more personalized approach that accommodates a variety of lifestyles. This chapter delves into how to adjust cannabis-infused meals to specific dietary needs, such as keto, paleo, vegan, and gluten-free. It also includes instructions for dosing and selecting strains based on desired health results and dietary constraints.

Tailoring Cannabis-Infused Meals for Individual Dietary Needs

Customizing cannabis-infused meals to meet certain dietary requirements, such as keto, paleo, vegan, and gluten-free, necessitates careful product selection and innovative cooking techniques. Here's a tip on how to customize cannabis-infused meals to your specific nutritional needs:

Keto-Friendly Cannabis Meals

Ingredients:

- Healthy fats, e.g., avocado, coconut oil, and ghee.
- Low-carb vegetables, e.g., spinach, kale, and cauliflower.
- Protein sources, e.g., salmon, eggs, and bacon.
- Cannabis-infused oils and butter.

Recipes:

CBD-infused avocado and bacon salad

THC-infused cauliflower mash

Cannabis-infused zucchini noodles with pesto.

Paleo-inspired Cannabis Dishes

Ingredients:

- Whole foods, e.g., lean meats, fish, nuts, seeds.
- Natural fats, e.g., olive oil, coconut oil.

- Fresh veggies and fruits.
- Coconut oil or ghee infused with cannabis.

Recipes:

- Cannabis-infused fish with veggies
- CBD-infused sweet potato fries
- THC-infused almond and coconut energy balls.

Vegan Cannabis Options

Ingredients:

- Plant-based proteins, e.g., tofu, tempeh, and legumes.
- Vegetables and fruits, e.g., broccoli, chickpeas, and berries.
- Healthy fats, e.g., avocado and almonds.
- Cannabis-infused olive or coconut oil.

Recipes:

- THC-infused chickpea stew
- CBD-infused quinoa salad

- Cannabis-infused coconut and berry smoothie.

Gluten-free Cannabis Recipes:

Ingredients:

- Gluten-free grains, e.g., quinoa and rice
- Gluten-free flours, e.g., almond and coconut flour.
- Vegetables and proteins, e.g., leafy greens, chicken, and fish.
- Cannabis-infused olive oil or butter.

Recipes:

- Cannabis-infused, gluten-free brownies
- CBD-infused vegetable stir-fry with rice
- THC-infused almond and coconut pancakes.

General Advice for Creating Cannabis-Infused Recipes

Dosage Control:

- Modify the cannabis dosage by personal tolerance and intended effects.
- Increase gradually after starting with smaller quantities.

Choose the Correct Strains:

- Take into account strains that have a balanced CBD and THC content or customize strains to support particular dietary objectives.
- Investigate terpenes for flavor enhancement and possible medical advantages.

Incorporate Infused Ingredients:

- Utilize tinctures, oils, or butter in recipes to achieve controlled dosages.
- Try a variety of infusion techniques according to the selected dietary plan.

Mindful Pairing:

- Match the tastes of cannabis strains to complement the entire dining experience.

- Consider complementing terpene profiles
  for the dish.

Experiment with Cooking Methods:

- Choose cooking methods that match your
  food choices, such as grilling, roasting, or
  sautéing.
- Adjust cooking times to maintain
  cannabinoids and terpenes.

Label and Record:

- Clearly label cannabis-infused items to
  minimize confusion.
- Record dosages and strain preferences for
  future reference.

Seek Professional Advice:

- Consult healthcare professionals or
  cannabis experts for personalized advice.
- Work with skilled cannabis chefs on
  advanced customization.

Guidelines for Dosing and Choosing Strains Based on Desired Health Goals and Dietary Restrictions

When introducing cannabis into meals, appropriate dosage and selection of strains are crucial, especially when desired health effects and dietary constraints are taken into account. Here are some important pointers to help with the process:

Recognize Individual Tolerance:

- Begin with a low dose and gradually raise it to get the right balance.
- Individual considerations to consider include metabolism, body weight, and cannabis experience.

Balanced CBD and THC:

- For a well-rounded experience, choose strains or products with a balanced CBD and THC concentration.

- CBD may provide therapeutic advantages while avoiding the strong euphoric effects associated with higher THC levels.

Customize Strains to Desired Effects:

- Sativa strains can be used during the day to give energy and focus.
- Indica strains are more typically linked to relaxation and are best used in the evening or before bed.
- Breeds that are hybrids blend traits from the two.

Examine Terpene Profiles:

- Terpenes add to cannabis's scent and effects.
- Myrcene may encourage calm, while limonene may provide an uplifting impact.
- Pinene may improve focus, whereas linalool may be relaxing.

Accurate Dosage in Infused Ingredients:

- When infusing oils or but, determine the overall cannabis dosage for the batch.
- To ensure consistent dosing, measure servings accurately.

Start Low, Go Slow:

- This is especially important for individuals new to cannabis or trying a new strain.
- Take time between doses to examine the effects before increasing.

Mindful Pairing with Dietary Restrictions:

- For keto or paleo diets, choose cannabis-infused oils like coconut or olive oil.
- Vegan recipes can use cannabis-infused plant-based oils or tinctures.
- Infused oils and gluten-free flours can be used in gluten-free recipes.

Experiment with Different Strains:

- Determine the optimal strains for certain health outcomes.
- Keep track of strains and their effects to guide future decisions.

Use Lab-Tested Products:

- Select cannabis products that have been tested for accurate cannabinoid content.
- Lab results include THC and CBD percentages, allowing for more exact dosing.

Consulting Professionals:

- Get personalized advice from healthcare or cannabis experts.
- Professional cannabis chefs can provide information on dose and strain pairing for culinary creations.

Take into Account Microdosing:

- Microdosing is the practice of ingesting tiny, regulated doses of cannabis to produce mild effects.

- This strategy can help control health outcomes without having unduly psychotic effects.

Label Infused Products:

- Label cannabis-infused products with dosages and strain details clearly and understandably;
- Keep infused products separate from ordinary ones to avoid inadvertent intake.

Legal Considerations:

- Follow local legislation and understand the legal implications of cannabis use in your location.

Appendix:

1. Guide for Dosing and Calculating the Potency of Homemade Cannabis Infusions.

Understanding potency and dose is critical for developing consistent and safe cannabis-infused foods. Here is an in-depth guide:

a. Calculating Cannabinoid Content:

- Determine the proportion of THC and CBD in the cannabis strain used.
- Multiply the percentage by the total weight of cannabis to calculate the total milligrams of THC and CBD.

b. Infusing Oils or Butters:

- Divide the THC or CBD sum in milligrams from the oil or butter volume.
- This gives the number of cannabinoids present in milligrams per milliliter or gram.

c. Serving Calculation:

- Split up the total milligrams by the required dosage per serving.
- This provides the quantity of servings, which makes exact dosage possible.

d. Consistent Mixing:

- Mix cannabis-infused ingredients evenly throughout the recipe for an accurate dose in each serving.

e. Modifying Dosage:

- Experiment with dosage to determine the ideal quantity for desired effects, taking into account each person's tolerance levels.

2. Safety Guidelines for Responsible and Legal Cannabis Consumption:

A positive cannabis experience requires responsible and legal cannabis intake. Follow these instructions:

a. Recognise Local Laws:

- Comply with applicable cannabis laws and regulations in your area.
- Respect the legal age restrictions and possession limitations.

b. Start Low, Go Slow:

- Start with minimal dosages, particularly if you're new to cannabis or trying a new strain.
- Give yourself plenty of time in between doses to gauge the effects before taking more.

c. Avoid Driving Under the Influence:

- Cannabis can impair coordination and response time.
- Avoid driving or using machinery while under the influence.

d. Keep Cannabis Goods Secure:

- Keep cannabis goods in a secure location, especially if there are children or pets in the household.

e. Clear Labeling:

- Label handmade cannabis-infused items with dose information.
- Please indicate whether the product contains THC, CBD, or a combination of the two.

f. Respect Others' Boundaries:

- Consider others' cannabis use preferences.
- Avoid consuming in public areas where it is forbidden.

g. Be Aware of Medical Issues:

- Whenever consuming cannabis, speak with a healthcare provider, especially if you have any pre-existing medical issues or are taking medication.

h. Avoid Combining with Alcohol or Other Substances:

- Combining cannabis with alcohol or certain drugs may intensify its effects.
- Use caution and understand potential interactions.

i. Seek Professional Advice:

- Speak to medical practitioners or cannabis professionals when worried concerning cannabis amount, strain choice, or any other element of its use.

j. Educate Yourself:

- Research the effects of various cannabinoids and terpenes.
- Practice responsible and safe cannabis use.

k. Responsible Cannabis Disposal:

- Discard unused or expired cannabis products.

- Follow local cannabis waste disposal guidelines.

Conclusion

To summarize, including cannabis in a health-conscious lifestyle can be a tasty and rewarding experience when conducted appropriately. As you explore the world of cannabis-infused meals meant to match varied dietary preferences and health goals, keep in mind the significance of mindfulness and making educated decisions.

Encouragement to Integrate Cannabis Responsibly:

Recognize the diversity of cannabis as a culinary element, including its ability to improve flavors, encourage relaxation, and contribute to overall health. Whether you're making infused salads, smoothies, or mindful snacks, cannabis may be a delicious addition to your health-conscious culinary adventures. Consult with healthcare professionals: When exploring cannabis for health and fitness, prioritize your well-being. Consulting with healthcare specialists guarantees that you receive personalized advice based on your specific health needs. Their experience can assist you in making informed decisions, particularly if you have pre-existing medical conditions or are researching cannabis for specific therapeutic objectives.

Embrace Balance: As you embark on your adventure, remember that balance is essential. Whether you want to use cannabis for relaxation, fitness rehabilitation, or overall well-being, choosing the correct strains, doses, and infusion methods is crucial.

Responsible Exploration: Celebrate cannabis' confluence with health and fitness in a responsible and informed way. Continue to educate yourself about the changing landscape of cannabis research, regulations, and best practices to make decisions that are consistent with your aims and values.

Incorporate cannabis into your daily life with inquiry, responsibility, and a commitment to overall wellness. May your cannabis-infused culinary excursions promote a balanced and gratifying approach to well-being.

Cheers to a careful, health-conscious cannabis adventure!